You Can Prevent and Heal Your Heart:

A Comprehensive Guide to Reversing Cardiovascular Disease for Individuals and Families

"Prevention is better than cure."

Introduction

Your heart is the engine of your life. It works tirelessly, day and night, to keep you going. But when this vital organ begins to falter, it can feel like the very foundation of your existence is crumbling. In You Can Prevent and Heal Your Heart, you'll discover a roadmap to rebuilding your cardiac health, brick by brick.

This book is more than just information; it's a beacon of hope, empowering individuals and families to reclaim their vitality and live life to the fullest.

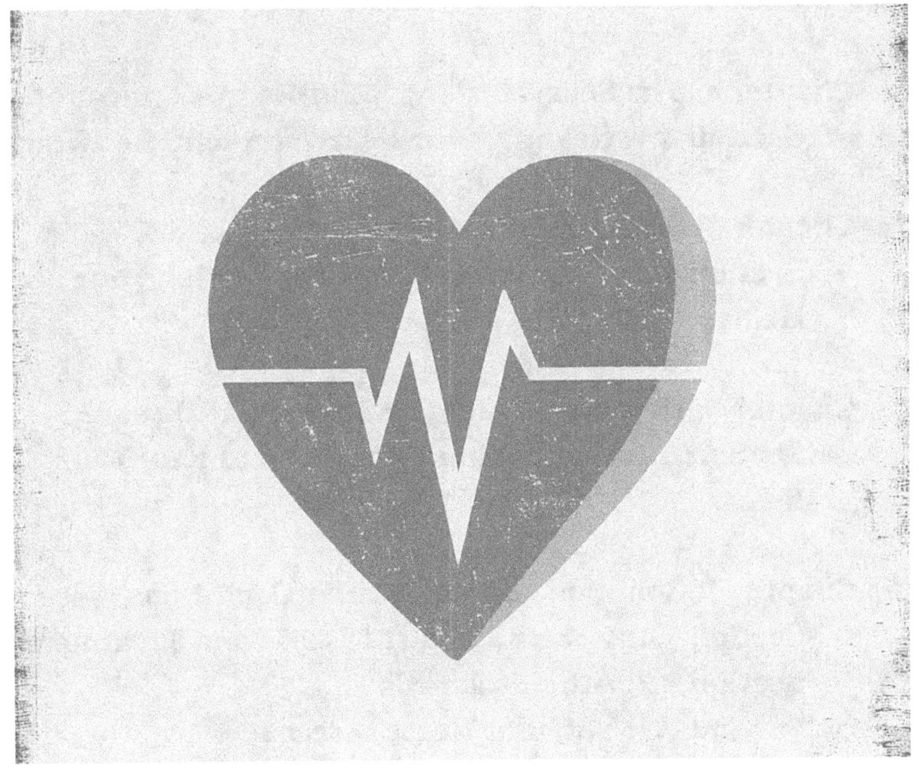

Contents

Contents

Contents

Part 1: Understanding Your Heart

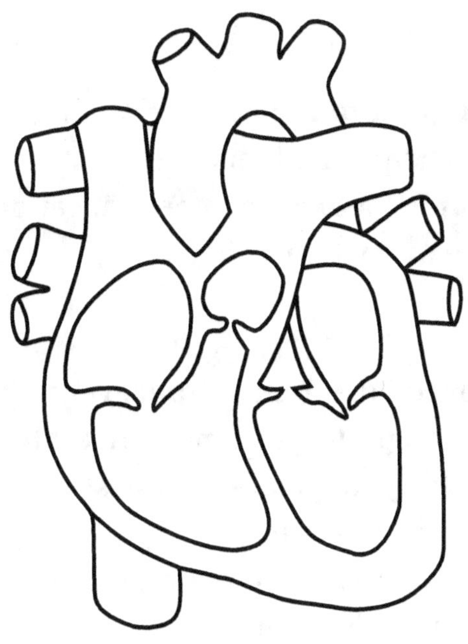

The foundation of cardiovascular health is built upon a complex interplay of genetic, environmental, and lifestyle factors. Understanding these foundational elements is crucial for preventing and managing heart disease.

Key Components

Genetics

- **Family history:** A strong family history of heart disease increases individual risk.
- **Genetic predispositions:** Certain genetic variations can influence heart health.

Environment

- **Exposure to pollutants:** Air and water pollution can contribute to heart problems.
- **Socioeconomic factors:** Income, education, and access to healthcare impact heart health.

Lifestyle

- **Diet:** A balanced diet rich in fruits, vegetables, whole grains, and lean proteins supports heart health.
- **Physical activity:** Regular exercise strengthens the heart and improves circulation.
- **Weight management:** Maintaining a healthy weight reduces strain on the heart.
- **Smoking:** Smoking damages blood vessels and increases heart disease risk.
- **Alcohol consumption:** Excessive alcohol intake can harm the heart.

- Sleep: Adequate sleep is essential for heart health.
- Stress management: Chronic stress can negatively impact the cardiovascular system.

Importance of Early Intervention

Building a strong foundation of cardiovascular health starts early in life. Preventive measures, such as healthy eating habits, regular exercise, and avoiding smoking, can significantly reduce the risk of heart disease later in life.

Additional Considerations

- **Chronic conditions:** Conditions like diabetes, high blood pressure, and high cholesterol are major risk factors for heart disease.
- **Regular check-ups:** Routine medical exams help identify and manage risk factors.

Overview

The heart is a complex muscular organ that acts as a pump, circulating blood throughout the body. Understanding its structure is essential to appreciate its function.

The Heart's Chambers

The heart is divided into four chambers:

- **Right atrium:** Receives oxygen-poor blood from the body.
- **Right ventricle:** Pumps oxygen-poor blood to the lungs.
- **Left atrium:** Receives oxygen-rich blood from the lungs.
- **Left ventricle:** Pumps oxygen-rich blood to the body.

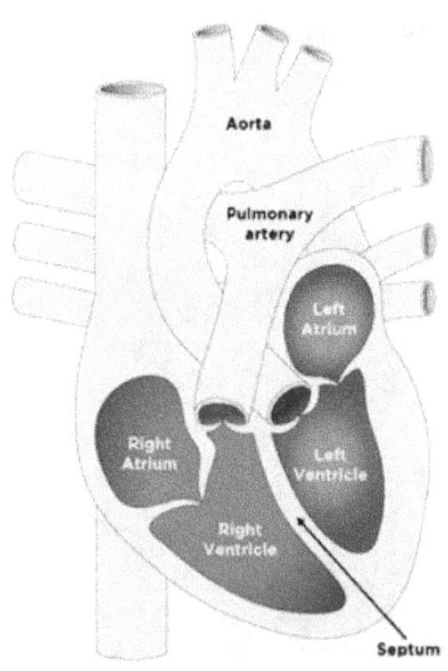

Heart Valves

Valves prevent blood from flowing backward. There are four main valves:

- **Tricuspid valve:** Located between the right atrium and right ventricle.
- **Pulmonary valve:** Located between the right ventricle and the pulmonary artery.
- **Mitral valve:** Located between the left atrium and left ventricle.
- **Aortic valve:** Located between the left ventricle and the aorta.

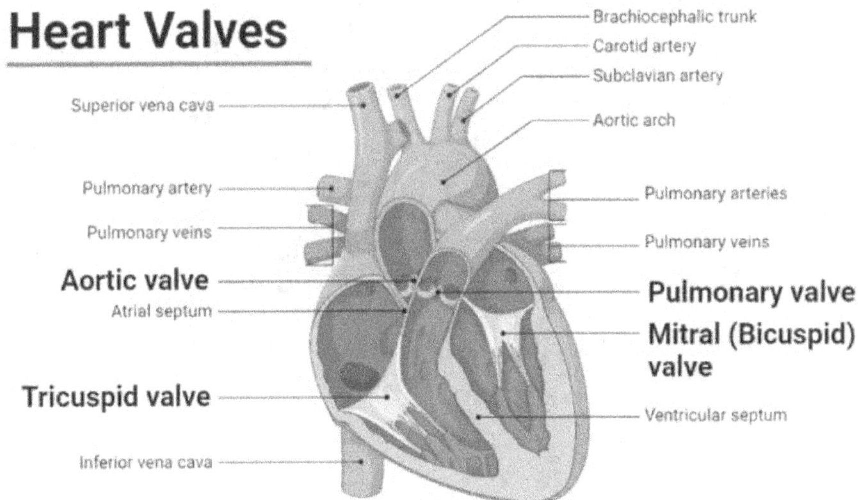

The Heart Wall

The heart wall consists of three layers:

- **Epicardium:** The outer layer.
- **Myocardium**: The thick middle layer composed of muscle.
- **Endocardium:** The inner layer lining the chambers.

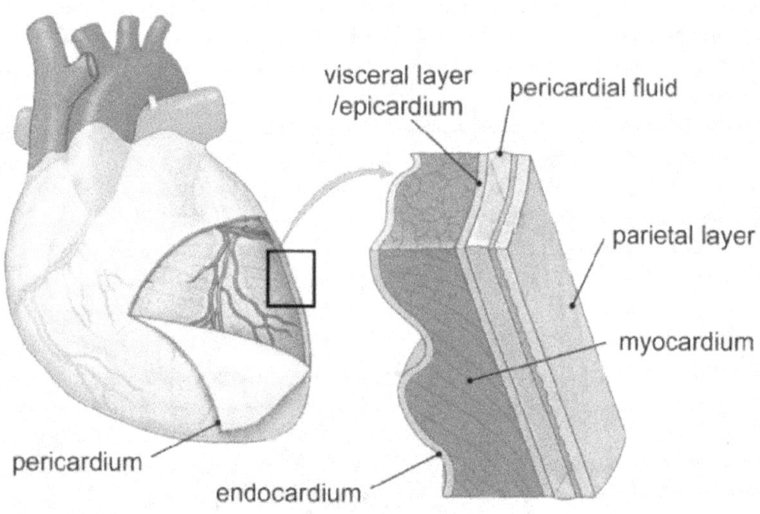

Blood Vessels

- **Coronary arteries:** Supply blood to the heart muscle itself.
- **Pulmonary artery:** Carries oxygen-poor blood to the lungs.
- **Pulmonary veins:** Return oxygen-rich blood from the lungs to the heart.
- **Aorta:** Carries oxygen-rich blood from the heart to the body.
- **Vena cava:** Returns oxygen-poor blood from the body to the heart.

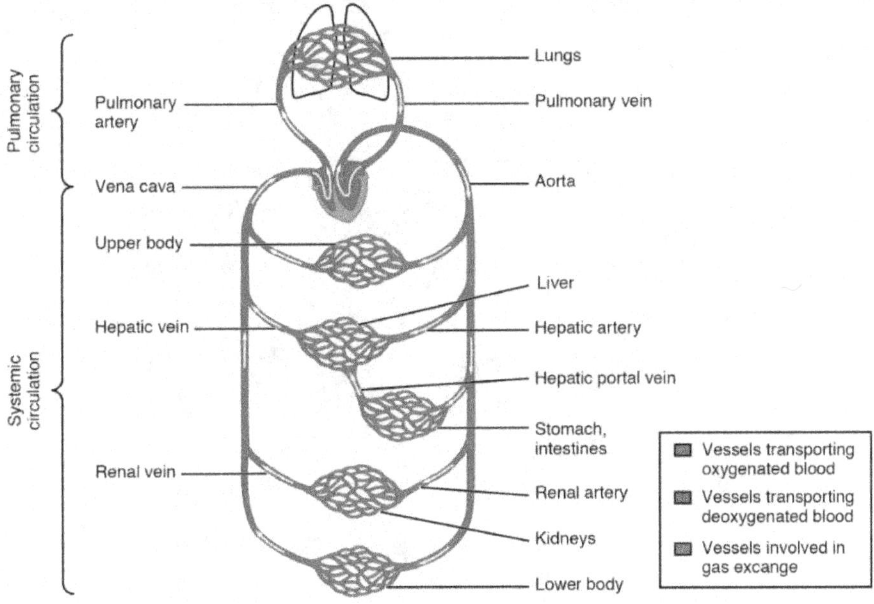

The Electrical System

The heart's electrical system controls its rhythm. Key components include:

- **Sinoatrial (SA) node:** The heart's natural pacemaker.
- **Atrioventricular (AV) node:** Conducts electrical signals from the atria to the ventricles.
- **Bundle of His and Purkinje fibers:** Distribute electrical signals throughout the ventricles.

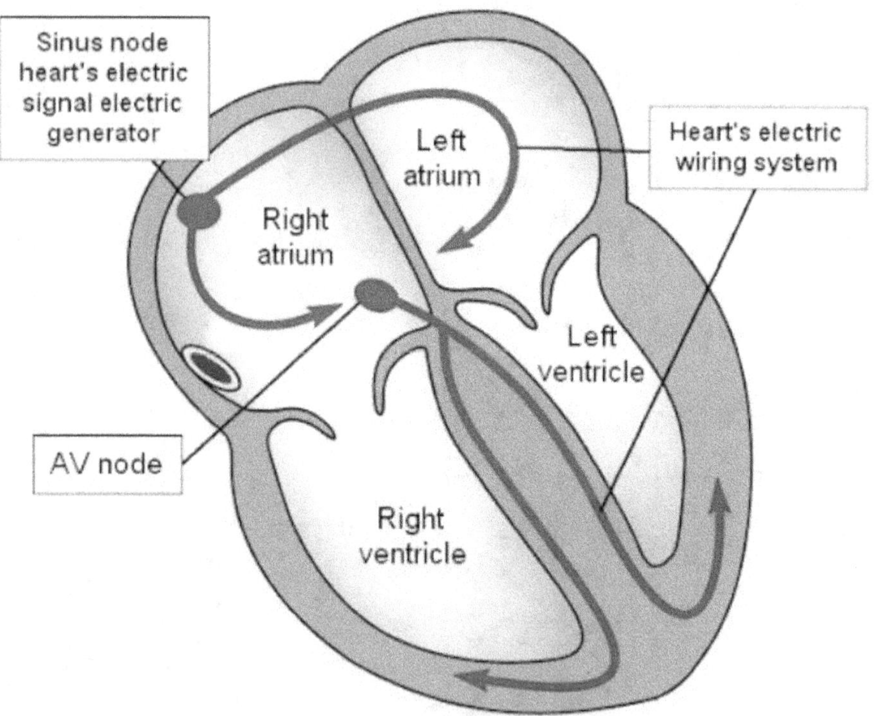

The heart is essentially a muscular pump that circulates blood throughout the body.

Key Functions:

- **Oxygen and nutrient delivery:** The heart pumps oxygen-rich blood from the lungs to the body's cells, providing the necessary nutrients for survival.

- **Waste removal:** It carries carbon dioxide and other waste products from the body's cells back to the lungs and kidneys for elimination.

- **Hormone transport:** The heart helps distribute hormones throughout the body, regulating various bodily functions.

- **Temperature regulation:** Blood circulation helps maintain a stable body temperature.

- **Immune system support:** White blood cells, crucial for fighting infections, are transported by the blood.

The Circulatory System

The heart is the central organ of the circulatory system, working in conjunction with blood vessels (arteries, veins, and capillaries) to achieve its functions.

The heart's primary function is to ensure efficient circulation of blood throughout the body. Blood is vital for delivering oxygen and nutrients to cells, removing waste products, and maintaining body temperature.

The Circulatory System

- Heart: The pump that propels blood.
- Blood vessels: A network of tubes carrying blood, including:
  - Arteries: Carry oxygenated blood away from the heart.
  - Veins: Carry deoxygenated blood back to the heart.
  - Capillaries: Tiny vessels where exchange of gases, nutrients, and waste occurs.

Blood Flow

- Pulmonary circulation: Blood travels from the heart to the lungs for oxygenation, then returns to the heart.
- Systemic circulation: Oxygenated blood is pumped from the heart to the body's tissues and organs, delivering oxygen and nutrients. Deoxygenated blood returns to the heart.

Factors Affecting Circulation

- Heart rate: The speed at which the heart beats.
- Blood pressure: The force exerted by blood against artery walls.
- Blood volume: The amount of blood circulating in the body.
- Blood vessel resistance: The opposition to blood flow.

Circulation and Overall Health

Efficient circulation is crucial for:

- Organ function: Adequate blood supply is essential for brain, kidney, liver, and other organ health.
- Wound healing: Blood carries necessary cells and nutrients for tissue repair.
- Temperature regulation: Blood helps maintain body temperature.
- Immune function: White blood cells, essential for fighting infection, are transported in blood.

Understanding the importance of circulation helps in maintaining overall health and preventing circulatory disorders.

Chapter 3: Importance of Circulation

Several factors can influence the efficiency of your circulation:

Lifestyle Factors:

- **Physical Activity:** Regular exercise, especially aerobic exercises like walking, swimming, or cycling, helps pump blood more efficiently.

- **Diet:** A balanced diet rich in fruits, vegetables, whole grains, and lean proteins supports heart health and blood vessel function.

- **Smoking:** Smoking damages blood vessels and increases the risk of blood clots, hindering circulation.

- **Alcohol Consumption:** Excessive alcohol consumption can harm the heart and blood vessels.

- **Stress:** Chronic stress can elevate blood pressure and contribute to circulatory problems.

Chapter 3: Importance of Circulation

Health Conditions:

- **Obesity**: Excess weight can put strain on the heart and contribute to high blood pressure and cholesterol.

- **Diabetes**: Uncontrolled diabetes can damage blood vessels.

- **Heart Disease:** Conditions like coronary artery disease can reduce blood flow to the heart.

- **Varicose Veins:** Weak or damaged veins can impair circulation in the legs.

Other Factors:

- **Medications**: Some medications can affect blood pressure or blood clotting.

- **Age**: As we age, blood vessels can become less elastic, affecting circulation.

By understanding these factors, you can take steps to improve your circulation and overall health.

Chapter 3: Importance of Circulation

Poor circulation, or reduced blood flow to the body's extremities, can manifest in several ways:

Common Symptoms:

- Cold hands and feet: This is often the first noticeable sign.

- Numbness or tingling: A pins-and-needles sensation, especially in the hands and feet.

- Pain: Aching or cramping in the muscles, particularly in the legs.

- Skin changes: Pale, blue, or red skin color, especially in the extremities.

- Weak or slow-healing wounds: Reduced blood flow hinders the healing process.

- Hair loss: In severe cases, hair loss can occur on the legs and feet.

- Fatigue: Lack of oxygen-rich blood can lead to tiredness.

More Serious Symptoms:

- Chest pain: If experienced along with other symptoms, it could indicate a heart problem.

- Swelling: In the legs or ankles, it might suggest circulatory issues.

- Dizziness or lightheadedness: Reduced blood flow to the brain can cause these symptoms.

It's important to note that these symptoms can be caused by various conditions, and it's essential to consult a healthcare professional for a proper diagnosis.

Part 2: Risk Factors and Conditions

The mind and heart are intricately connected, forming a complex bidirectional relationship. This connection significantly impacts our overall health and well-being.

The Mind-Heart Connection

- **Neurological Connection:** The heart and brain communicate through a vast network of nerves. The heart even has its own intrinsic nervous system, often referred to as the "brain of the heart."

- **Hormonal Influence:** Hormones released by the heart, such as atrial natriuretic peptide (ANP), influence blood pressure and fluid balance. Additionally, stress hormones like cortisol can impact heart health.

- **Electromagnetic Field:** The heart generates the most potent electromagnetic field in the body, which can influence brain activity and emotional states.

Healing Your Heart Through the Mind

- Stress Management: Chronic stress negatively impacts heart health. Techniques like meditation, deep breathing, and yoga can help manage stress and its effects on the cardiovascular system.

- Positive Emotions: Cultivating positive emotions, such as gratitude, compassion, and joy, has been linked to improved heart health.

- Mindfulness: Being present in the moment can reduce stress and anxiety, promoting heart health.

- Biofeedback: This technique helps individuals learn to control physiological responses, including heart rate and blood pressure.

The Power of the Mind-Body Connection

By understanding the intricate relationship between the mind and heart, we can harness the power of our thoughts and emotions to promote cardiovascular health. Incorporating mind-body practices into daily life can significantly contribute to overall well-being.

Meditation for Heart Health

Meditation is a cornerstone of mind-body medicine for heart health. It involves training your mind to focus and redirect your thoughts.

- Benefits: Reduces stress, lowers blood pressure, and improves heart rate variability.

- Techniques: There are various meditation techniques, including mindfulness meditation, transcendental meditation, and loving-kindness meditation.

Biofeedback: Gaining Control

Biofeedback is a technique that helps you become aware of your physiological responses, such as heart rate, blood pressure, and muscle tension. With practice, you can learn to control these responses.

- Benefits: Can lower blood pressure, reduce stress, and improve heart rate variability.

- Applications: Used in managing conditions like anxiety and hypertension.

Cognitive-Behavioral Therapy (CBT)

CBT focuses on identifying and changing negative thought patterns and behaviors. It can be effective in managing stress and anxiety, which positively impact heart health.

- Benefits: Helps reduce stress, improve mood, and promote heart-healthy behaviors.

- Applications: Useful for conditions like depression and anxiety, which often accompany heart problems.

Other Mind-Body Techniques

- Yoga: Combines physical postures, breathing exercises, and meditation. It can lower stress and improve cardiovascular health.

- Tai Chi: Gentle exercises and meditation promote relaxation and balance.

- Hypnosis: Can help manage pain, reduce anxiety, and improve sleep, all of which benefit heart health.

Remember, incorporating these practices into your daily life can have a profound impact on your heart health. It's essential to consult with a healthcare professional before starting any new wellness program.

Stress is a common aspect of modern life, but chronic stress can have a detrimental impact on heart health. When the body perceives stress, it initiates a "fight-or-flight" response, leading to physiological changes like increased heart rate, blood pressure, and cortisol levels.

How Stress Affects the Heart

- Increased Heart Rate and Blood Pressure: Chronic stress can lead to sustained high blood pressure, a major risk factor for heart disease, stroke, and heart failure.

- Cortisol and Inflammation: Prolonged stress elevates cortisol levels, which can contribute to inflammation throughout the body, including the heart.

- Unhealthy Coping Mechanisms: Stress often leads to unhealthy behaviors like smoking, overeating, and decreased physical activity, all of which increase heart disease risk.

- Weakened Immune System: Chronic stress can suppress the immune system, making you more susceptible to infections that can exacerbate heart problems.

Controlling Stress for Heart Health

- Identify Stressors: Recognizing the sources of stress is the first step towards managing them.

- Time Management: Effective time management can help reduce feelings of overwhelm.

- Relaxation Techniques: Practices like meditation, deep breathing, and yoga can activate the body's relaxation response.

- Regular Exercise: Physical activity helps reduce stress and improves overall cardiovascular health.

- Sufficient Sleep: Adequate sleep is essential for stress management and heart health.

- Social Support: Strong social connections can buffer the effects of stress.

- Healthy Lifestyle: A balanced diet, regular exercise, and avoiding smoking and excessive alcohol consumption contribute to overall well-being and stress management.

By implementing these strategies, you can significantly reduce the negative impact of stress on your heart and improve your overall cardiovascular health.

Depression and heart disease share a complex relationship. Not only can depression increase the risk of developing heart problems, but it can also worsen the prognosis for those already living with heart disease. Understanding this connection is crucial for effective heart health management.

The Link Between Depression and Heart Disease

- Shared Risk Factors: Many factors contribute to both depression and heart disease, including stress, unhealthy lifestyle choices, and genetics.

- Biological Overlap: Both conditions involve imbalances in neurotransmitters and hormones.

- Behavioral Changes: Depression can lead to unhealthy behaviors like decreased physical activity, poor diet, and increased smoking or alcohol consumption, which further impact heart health.

Controlling Depression to Heal Your Heart

Addressing depression is a vital component of heart health care.

- Open Communication: Talk to your healthcare provider about your feelings and concerns.

- Medication: Antidepressants may be prescribed to help manage symptoms.

- Therapy: Cognitive-behavioral therapy (CBT) can help you identify and change negative thought patterns.

- Lifestyle Changes: Regular exercise, a healthy diet, and adequate sleep can improve mood and overall well-being.

- Support Groups: Connecting with others who understand your experience can be beneficial.

Remember, seeking help for depression is a sign of strength, not weakness. By addressing both physical and mental health, you can significantly improve your heart health and quality of life.

Depression and heart disease are intricately linked, forming a vicious cycle that can significantly impact quality of life. Understanding this connection is essential for effective management.

The Impact of Depression on Heart Health

- Increased Risk Factors: Depression often coincides with other heart disease risk factors, such as smoking, unhealthy diet, and lack of exercise.

- Inflammation: Depressive symptoms can trigger inflammatory responses in the body, contributing to heart disease.

- Adherence to Treatment: Depression can make it difficult to follow heart-healthy treatment plans, such as medication and lifestyle changes.

- Increased Risk of Heart Events: Studies have shown that individuals with depression are at a higher risk of heart attacks and strokes.

The Impact of Heart Disease on Depression

- Lifestyle Changes: The adjustments required to manage heart disease can lead to feelings of isolation and depression.

- Fear and Anxiety: The fear of future heart problems can contribute to anxiety and depression.

- Physical Limitations: Heart disease symptoms can limit physical activity and social interactions, leading to feelings of isolation.

The Role of Social Support

Social connections play a vital role in managing both depression and heart disease.

- Emotional Support: Talking to friends, family, or a support group can help alleviate feelings of loneliness and isolation.

- Practical Support: Having people to rely on for assistance with daily tasks can reduce stress.

- Accountability: Support systems can help individuals stick to treatment plans and healthy lifestyle changes.

By prioritizing mental health and seeking support, individuals can improve their overall well-being and reduce the risk of heart-related complications.

Ischemic heart disease occurs when the heart muscle isn't receiving enough blood. This typically happens due to a blockage in the coronary arteries, the vessels supplying blood to the heart.

Causes

- Atherosclerosis: A buildup of fatty substances (plaque) in the coronary arteries.
- Coronary artery spasm: Temporary narrowing of the coronary arteries.
- Coronary embolism: A blood clot blocking a coronary artery.

Symptoms

Symptoms can vary based on severity. Common ones include:

- Chest pain (angina): Often described as a squeezing or pressure.
- Shortness of breath
- Fatigue
- Dizziness
- Heart palpitations

Types

- Stable angina: Chest pain triggered by exertion, relieved by rest or medication.
- Unstable angina: Chest pain at rest or with minimal effort, often a precursor to a heart attack.
- Heart attack: Complete blockage of blood flow to a part of the heart, causing heart muscle damage.

Treatment

Treatment for ischemic heart disease focuses on relieving symptoms, preventing heart attacks, and improving overall heart health.

Medications

Medications are often the first line of treatment:

- Nitrates: These relax blood vessels, providing temporary relief from chest pain (angina).
- Beta-blockers: These slow down the heart rate and reduce blood pressure, decreasing the heart's workload.
- Calcium channel blockers: These relax blood vessels and reduce heart muscle contraction.
- Statins: These lower cholesterol levels to prevent plaque buildup in arteries.
- Aspirin: This helps prevent blood clots.
- ACE inhibitors and ARBs: These manage blood pressure and protect the heart.

Procedures

When medications aren't enough, procedures may be considered:

- Angioplasty and Stenting: A balloon is inflated to open a blocked artery, and a stent is often placed to keep it open.

- Coronary Artery Bypass Surgery (CABG): This involves creating new pathways for blood to flow around blocked arteries.

Lifestyle Changes

Lifestyle modifications are crucial for managing ischemic heart disease:

- Healthy Diet: Low in saturated and trans fats, rich in fruits, vegetables, and whole grains.
- Regular Exercise: Improves heart health and helps manage weight.
- Weight Management: Being overweight increases the risk of heart disease.
- Smoking Cessation: Smoking damages blood vessels.
- Stress Management: Reduces the heart's workload.

It's important to work closely with your doctor to determine the best treatment plan for you.

Atherosclerosis is a condition where plaque builds up inside your arteries. This plaque is made of fat, cholesterol, and other substances. Over time, it hardens and narrows your arteries, reducing blood flow.

How it Happens

- Plaque buildup: Cholesterol, fat, and other substances stick to artery walls, forming plaque.
- Artery narrowing: Plaque makes arteries narrower, restricting blood flow.
- Blood clot risk: Plaque can rupture, leading to a blood clot that can block the artery completely.

Risk Factors

- High blood pressure
- High cholesterol
- Smoking
- Diabetes
- Obesity
- Lack of exercise
- Unhealthy diet
- Family history

Complications

Atherosclerosis can lead to serious problems:
- Heart attack
- Stroke
- Peripheral artery disease
- Aortic aneurysm

Preventing and Treating Atherosclerosis

Prevention

Atherosclerosis often starts early in life, so prevention is key:

- Healthy Diet: Focus on fruits, vegetables, whole grains, lean proteins, and healthy fats. Limit saturated and trans fats, cholesterol, sodium, and added sugars.

- Regular Exercise: Aim for at least 30 minutes of moderate-intensity exercise most days of the week.

- Weight Management: Maintain a healthy weight to reduce strain on the heart.

- Quit Smoking: Smoking significantly increases the risk of atherosclerosis.

- Manage Stress: Find healthy ways to cope with stress, such as meditation or yoga.

- Regular Check-ups: Monitor blood pressure, cholesterol, and blood sugar levels.

Treatment

Treatment depends on the severity of atherosclerosis:

- Medications:Statins: Lower cholesterol levels.
- Blood pressure medications: Control high blood pressure.
- Aspirin: Helps prevent blood clots.
- Other medications as needed.

- Lifestyle Changes: The same as prevention, but with a stronger emphasis on adherence.

  - Procedures:Angioplasty and stenting: To open blocked arteries.
  - Coronary artery bypass surgery: In severe cases.

Early detection and treatment are crucial. Working closely with your doctor is essential for developing a personalized plan.

Valvular heart disease happens when the heart's valves don't work properly. These valves control blood flow through the heart.

Types of Valve Problems

- Stenosis: The valve opening narrows, making it harder for blood to flow through.
- Regurgitation: The valve doesn't close tightly, allowing blood to leak backward.
- Prolapse: The valve flaps bulge into the heart chamber.

Causes

- Born with it: Some people are born with abnormal valves.
- Infections: Like endocarditis, which can damage valves.
- Rheumatic fever: A condition that can damage heart valves.
- Wear and tear: Valves can become damaged over time.

Symptoms

Symptoms can vary but might include:

- Shortness of breath
- Chest pain
- Fatigue
- Irregular heartbeat
- Swelling in legs or ankles

Preventing Valvular Heart Disease

While some cases of valvular heart disease are congenital, others can be prevented or managed through:

- Early Treatment of Infections: Promptly treating infections like strep throat can help prevent rheumatic fever, a leading cause of valve damage.

- Healthy Lifestyle: Maintaining a healthy weight, exercising regularly, and eating a balanced diet can reduce the risk of heart disease in general.

- Regular Check-ups: Regular medical examinations can help detect early signs of valve problems.

Treatment for valvular heart disease aims to manage symptoms, prevent complications, and improve heart function.

Medications

- Diuretics: Help reduce fluid buildup, often causing swelling in legs and ankles.
- Digoxin: Strengthens the heart's contractions, improving its efficiency.
- Blood thinners: Prevent blood clots, reducing the risk of stroke.
- Antibiotics: Prevent endocarditis, an infection of the heart valves.

Surgical Interventions

For severe cases, surgery might be necessary:

- Valve Repair: Fixing the damaged valve to restore its function.

- Valve Replacement: Replacing the damaged valve with a mechanical or tissue valve.

- TAVR (Transcatheter Aortic Valve Replacement): A less invasive procedure to replace the aortic valve.

Lifestyle Changes

While not a direct treatment, these changes can significantly improve heart health:

- Regular Exercise: Strengthens the heart and improves circulation.
- Healthy Diet: Low in sodium, saturated fats, and cholesterol.
- Weight Management: Reduces strain on the heart.
- Quit Smoking: Improves overall heart health.
- Stress Management: Helps regulate heart rate and blood pressure.

Remember, it's essential to work closely with your doctor to determine the best treatment plan for your specific condition.

Heart failure occurs when your heart can't pump enough blood to meet your body's needs. It's often called congestive heart failure, but the term "heart failure" is more accurate. It doesn't mean your heart has stopped working, but rather that it's not working as efficiently as it should.

Causes

Many things can cause heart failure, including:

- Heart attacks
- High blood pressure
- Weakened heart muscle
- Valve problems

Symptoms

Heart failure symptoms can vary but often include:

- Shortness of breath
- Fatigue
- Weakness
- Swelling in legs, ankles, or feet
- Rapid or irregular heartbeat
- Coughing or wheezing
- Difficulty concentrating

Preventing Heart Failure

Many cases of heart failure can be prevented by addressing underlying conditions and adopting a heart-healthy lifestyle.

Key Prevention Strategies:

- Manage Chronic Conditions: Effectively control conditions like high blood pressure, diabetes, and high cholesterol.

- Healthy Diet: Focus on fruits, vegetables, whole grains, and lean proteins. Limit saturated and unhealthy fats, sodium, and added sugars.

- Regular Exercise: Aim for at least 30 minutes of moderate-intensity exercise most days of the week to strengthen the heart and improve circulation.

- Maintain a Healthy Weight: Being overweight can strain the heart.

- Don't Smoke: Smoking damages blood vessels and increases the risk of heart disease.

- Limit Alcohol: Excessive alcohol consumption can harm the heart.

- Manage Stress: Chronic stress can contribute to heart problems.

- Regular Check-ups: Monitor blood pressure, cholesterol, and blood sugar levels regularly.

By adopting these preventive measures, you can significantly reduce your risk of developing heart failure.

Treating Heart Failure

Heart failure treatment aims to manage symptoms, improve heart function, and prevent complications.

Medications

Medications are a cornerstone of heart failure treatment:

- Diuretics: Help reduce fluid buildup, easing swelling.
- ACE inhibitors and ARBs: Relax blood vessels, reducing the heart's workload.
- Beta-blockers: Slow heart rate and lower blood pressure.
- Digoxin: Strengthens heart contractions.
- Aldosterone antagonists: Reduce fluid retention.
- Other medications: May be used depending on specific needs.

Lifestyle Changes

Lifestyle plays a crucial role in managing heart failure:

- Diet: Low-sodium diet to reduce fluid buildup.
- Exercise: Regular physical activity improves heart health.
- Weight management: Can reduce strain on the heart.
- Quit smoking: Improves overall heart health.
- Stress management: Helps regulate heart rate and blood pressure.

Medical Devices

In some cases, medical devices can assist heart function:

- Pacemakers: Help regulate heart rhythm.
- Implantable defibrillators: Prevent dangerous heart rhythms.
- Ventricular assist devices (VADs): Support heart function as a bridge to transplant or long-term therapy.

Surgery

For severe cases, surgery might be considered:
- Heart transplant: Replacing the failing heart with a donor heart.
- Valve repair or replacement: If valve problems contribute to heart failure.

It's essential to work closely with your doctor to determine the best treatment plan.

Cardiomyopathy is a term for diseases that affect the heart muscle. These diseases can weaken the heart's ability to pump blood effectively, leading to heart failure.

Types of Cardiomyopathy

There are several types of cardiomyopathy, each with its own characteristics:

- Dilated cardiomyopathy: The heart's chambers become enlarged and weakened.

- Hypertrophic cardiomyopathy: The heart muscle becomes abnormally thick, making it harder for the heart to pump blood.

- Restrictive cardiomyopathy: The heart muscle becomes stiff, making it difficult for the heart to fill with blood.

- Arrhythmogenic right ventricular cardiomyopathy: This rare condition affects the heart's right ventricle, increasing the risk of irregular heartbeats.

Symptoms

Symptoms of cardiomyopathy can vary depending on the type and severity of the condition. Common symptoms include:

- Shortness of breath
- Fatigue
- Swelling in the legs, ankles, or feet
- Irregular heartbeat
- Dizziness or fainting

Causes

Cardiomyopathies can be caused by various factors, including:

- Genetic conditions
- Heart attacks
- High blood pressure
- Infections
- Alcohol abuse
- Certain medications
- Certain medications

Preventing Cardiomyopathies

While some types of cardiomyopathy are inherited and cannot be prevented, many can be reduced by adopting a heart-healthy lifestyle.

Key Prevention Strategies:

- Manage Underlying Conditions: Effectively control conditions like high blood pressure, diabetes, and high cholesterol.

- Healthy Diet: Consume a balanced diet rich in fruits, vegetables, whole grains, and lean proteins. Limit saturated and unhealthy fats, sodium, and added sugars.

- Regular Exercise: Aim for at least 30 minutes of moderate-intensity exercise most days of the week.

- Maintain a Healthy Weight: Obesity can strain the heart.

- Avoid Smoking and Excessive Alcohol: Both can damage the heart.

- Regular Check-ups: Monitor blood pressure, cholesterol, and blood sugar levels regularly.

- Genetic Counseling: If there's a family history of cardiomyopathy, consider genetic counseling.

By addressing these factors, you can significantly reduce your risk of developing cardiomyopathy.

Treating Cardiomyopathies

Treatment for cardiomyopathy depends on the specific type, its severity, and the underlying cause. The goal is to manage symptoms, improve heart function, and prevent complications.

General Treatment Approaches

- Medications: These are often the first line of treatment. They can help manage symptoms like shortness of breath, reduce the heart's workload, and regulate heart rhythm.

- Lifestyle Changes: Maintaining a healthy weight, regular exercise, and a balanced diet can improve heart health.

- Device Therapy: Implantable devices like pacemakers or defibrillators can help regulate heart rhythm and improve heart function.

- Surgery: In severe cases, surgery might be considered, such as heart transplantation or procedures to correct structural heart problems.

Specific Treatments Based on Cardiomyopathy Type

- Dilated Cardiomyopathy: Focuses on managing heart failure symptoms, improving heart function, and preventing complications. Medications, lifestyle changes, and device therapy are common treatments.

- Hypertrophic Cardiomyopathy: Aims to reduce the thickness of the heart muscle and improve blood flow. Medications, septal ablation (a minimally invasive procedure), or surgery (septal myectomy) might be considered.

- Restrictive Cardiomyopathy: Treatment often focuses on managing symptoms, as there are limited treatment options. Medications, heart transplantation, or surgery to remove scar tissue might be considered in some cases.

- Arrhythmogenic Right Ventricular Cardiomyopathy: Treatment involves managing heart rhythm disturbances, preventing sudden cardiac death, and reducing the risk of heart failure. Medications, implantable defibrillators, and surgery might be necessary.

It's crucial to work closely with a cardiologist to develop a personalized treatment plan.

Hypertension is a condition where the blood pressure in your arteries is consistently too high. It's often called the "silent killer" because it usually doesn't cause symptoms until it reaches a severe stage.

Understanding Blood Pressure

Blood pressure is measured in two numbers:

- Systolic pressure: The top number, which measures the pressure in your arteries when your heart beats.
- Diastolic pressure: The bottom number, which measures the pressure in your arteries when your heart rests between beats.

A blood pressure reading of 120/80 mmHg or lower is considered normal. Hypertension is diagnosed when your blood pressure is consistently 130/80 mmHg or higher.

Causes of Hypertension

In most cases, the exact cause of hypertension is unknown (primary hypertension). However, certain factors can contribute to it, including:

- Obesity
- Lack of physical activity
- Unhealthy diet
- Smoking
- Excessive alcohol consumption
- Stress
- Family history
- Age

- Certain medical conditions (kidney disease, thyroid problems)

Risks of Hypertension

Untreated hypertension can lead to serious health problems, such as:

- Heart attack
- Stroke
- Heart failure
- Kidney damage
- Vision problems

Preventing Hypertension

Preventing hypertension is largely about adopting a healthy lifestyle. Here are some key steps:

Lifestyle Modifications:

- Maintain a healthy weight: Being overweight or obese increases the risk of hypertension.
- Regular physical activity: Aim for at least 150 minutes of moderate-intensity exercise per week.
- Healthy diet: Focus on fruits, vegetables, whole grains, lean proteins, and low-fat dairy. Reduce sodium intake.
- Limit alcohol: Excessive alcohol consumption can raise blood pressure.
- Quit smoking: Smoking damages blood vessels and increases blood pressure.
- Manage stress: Chronic stress can contribute to hypertension.

- Adequate sleep: Lack of sleep can affect blood pressure regulation.

Regular Check-ups:
- Monitor your blood pressure regularly, especially if you have risk factors.
- Early detection allows for timely intervention.

Addressing Underlying Conditions:
- Manage conditions like diabetes, sleep apnea, and kidney disease, as they can contribute to hypertension.

By incorporating these habits into your daily life, you can significantly reduce your risk of developing hypertension and improve your overall health.

Treating Hypertension

Treatment for hypertension typically involves a combination of lifestyle modifications and medications. The goal is to lower blood pressure to a healthy level to reduce the risk of heart disease, stroke, and other complications.

Lifestyle Changes:

- Weight management: Losing even a small amount of weight can significantly lower blood pressure.

- Regular exercise: Aim for at least 150 minutes of moderate-intensity exercise per week.

- Dietary changes: Reduce sodium intake, increase potassium intake, and focus on fruits, vegetables, whole grains, and lean proteins.

- Limit alcohol: Excessive alcohol consumption can raise blood pressure.

- Quit smoking: Smoking damages blood vessels and increases blood pressure.

- Stress management: Practice relaxation techniques like meditation or yoga.

- Adequate sleep: Aim for 7-9 hours of quality sleep per night.

Medications:

If lifestyle changes alone aren't enough to control blood pressure, your doctor may prescribe medications. Common types include:

- Diuretics: Help remove excess fluid from the body.
- Angiotensin-converting enzyme (ACE) inhibitors: Relax blood vessels.
- Angiotensin II receptor blockers (ARBs): Also relax blood vessels.
- Beta-blockers: Slow heart rate and reduce blood pressure.
- Calcium channel blockers: Relax blood vessels and slow heart rate.
- Combination drugs: May be used for more severe hypertension.

It's important to take your medications as prescribed and monitor your blood pressure regularly.

Peripheral vascular disease (PVD) is a circulatory disorder that occurs when blood vessels become narrowed, blocked, or spasmed. This reduces blood flow to your limbs, often your legs and feet.

Causes of PVD

The most common cause of PVD is atherosclerosis, a buildup of plaque in the arteries. Other causes include blood clots, inflammation, and muscle spasms.

Symptoms of PVD

Symptoms can vary depending on the severity of the condition. Common symptoms include:

- Leg pain when walking (claudication)
- Numbness or coldness in the legs
- Weak pulse in the legs or feet
- Sores on the legs or feet that heal slowly
- Hair loss on the legs
- Changes in nail color
- Erectile dysfunction (in men)

Risk Factors for PVD

- Smoking
- High blood pressure
- High cholesterol
- Diabetes
- Obesity
- Older age

Preventing Peripheral Vascular Disease (PVD)

Preventing PVD often involves managing underlying health conditions and adopting a heart-healthy lifestyle.
Key Prevention Strategies:

- Manage Chronic Conditions: Effectively control conditions like high blood pressure, diabetes, and high cholesterol.

- Quit Smoking: Smoking is a major risk factor for PVD.
- Healthy Diet: Consume a diet rich in fruits, vegetables, whole grains, and lean proteins.

- Regular Exercise: Aim for at least 30 minutes of moderate-intensity exercise most days of the week.

- Maintain a Healthy Weight: Obesity increases the risk of PVD.

- Manage Stress: Chronic stress can contribute to heart health issues.

- Regular Check-ups: Monitor blood pressure, cholesterol, and blood sugar levels regularly.

By incorporating these habits into your daily life, you can significantly reduce your risk of developing PVD.

Treating Peripheral Vascular Disease (PVD)

Treatment for PVD aims to improve blood flow to the limbs, relieve symptoms, and prevent complications.

Lifestyle Changes

Lifestyle modifications are crucial for managing PVD:

- Regular Exercise: Helps improve blood flow to the legs.
- Quit Smoking: Smoking significantly damages blood vessels.
- Healthy Diet: Low in saturated fats, cholesterol, and sodium.
- Weight Management: Can reduce strain on the heart and improve circulation.
- Diabetes Management: Controlling blood sugar levels is essential.

Medications

Medications can help improve blood flow and prevent complications:

- Antiplatelet drugs: Prevent blood clots.
- Statins: Lower cholesterol levels.
- Blood pressure medications: Manage high blood pressure.
- Medications to improve blood flow: Can help relieve leg pain.

Medical Procedures

In more severe cases, procedures may be necessary:

- Angioplasty and stenting: To open blocked arteries.
- Bypass surgery: To reroute blood flow around blocked arteries.
- Endarterectomy: Removal of plaque from an artery.
- Amputation: In severe cases where the limb is not salvageable.

It's important to work closely with your healthcare provider to determine the best treatment plan for you.

For many years, cholesterol has been vilified as the primary culprit behind heart disease. While it's true that high cholesterol levels can contribute to heart disease, the relationship is more complex than often portrayed.

Understanding Cholesterol

Cholesterol is a waxy, fat-like substance found in all cells of the body. It's essential for producing hormones, vitamin D, and bile acid. There are two main types of cholesterol:

- Low-density lipoprotein (LDL): Often referred to as "bad" cholesterol, high levels can contribute to plaque buildup in arteries.

- High-density lipoprotein (HDL): Often referred to as "good" cholesterol, it helps remove LDL from the bloodstream.

The Cholesterol Myth

While it's important to manage LDL cholesterol levels, focusing solely on cholesterol can be misleading. Other factors play a significant role in heart health, including:

- Inflammation: Chronic inflammation is linked to heart disease, even in people with normal cholesterol levels.
- Blood sugar control: Diabetes is a major risk factor for heart disease.
- Blood pressure: High blood pressure damages arteries.

- Lifestyle factors: Smoking, obesity, and lack of exercise increase heart disease risk.

A Balanced Approach

Rather than obsessing over cholesterol numbers, it's essential to focus on overall heart health. This includes:

- Healthy diet: Rich in fruits, vegetables, whole grains, and lean proteins.
- Regular exercise: Helps control weight and blood pressure.
- Quitting smoking: Damages blood vessels.
- Managing stress: Can contribute to heart health.
- Regular check-ups: Monitor blood pressure, cholesterol, and blood sugar levels.

By adopting a holistic approach to heart health, you can significantly reduce your risk of heart disease, even if your cholesterol levels aren't perfect.

Superfoods for a Healthy Heart: Breakfast

Starting your day with a heart-healthy breakfast is crucial for overall well-being. Here are some superfood options to consider:

Oatmeal

Oatmeal is a fantastic breakfast choice for heart health. It's packed with soluble fiber, which helps lower cholesterol levels.

- Enhance your oatmeal with:Berries: Rich in antioxidants and fiber.
- Nuts and seeds: Provide healthy fats and protein.
- Chia seeds: Offer omega-3 fatty acids and fiber.

Greek Yogurt

Greek yogurt is a great source of protein and calcium, both essential for heart health.

- Combine with:Fresh fruits: Add sweetness and antioxidants.
- Nuts and seeds: For healthy fats and crunch.
- Honey: A natural sweetener (in moderation).

Avocado Toast

Avocado is rich in heart-healthy monounsaturated fats. Pair it with whole-grain bread for a satisfying and nutritious

breakfast.
- Enhance your toast with:A sprinkle of red pepper flakes: Adds flavor and may help reduce inflammation.
- A drizzle of olive oil: Another source of healthy fats.

Eggs

Eggs are a good source of protein and healthy fats. However, it's essential to consume them in moderation.

- Prepare your eggs:Poached or boiled are healthier options than fried.
- Combine with whole-grain toast and avocado for a balanced meal.

Remember:

- Portion control: Even healthy foods should be consumed in moderation.
- Variety: Incorporate different foods into your breakfast routine to ensure you're getting a wide range of nutrients.
- Hydration: Start your day with a glass of water.

By choosing heart-healthy breakfast options, you're taking a significant step towards improving your overall cardiovascular health.

Salads are a versatile and nutritious option for a heart-healthy meal. Packed with vitamins, minerals, and fiber, they can be customized to suit various tastes and dietary needs.

Key Ingredients for Heart-Healthy Salads

- Base: Opt for leafy greens like spinach, romaine, or arugula.
- Protein: Incorporate lean protein sources like grilled chicken, fish, tofu, or beans.
- Healthy fats: Add avocados, nuts, or seeds for heart-healthy fats and flavor.
- Fiber: Include plenty of vegetables and whole grains for added fiber.
- Antioxidants: Incorporate colorful fruits and vegetables for their antioxidant properties.

Salad Dressing Ideas

- Homemade dressings: Use olive oil, lemon juice, vinegar, and herbs for a healthier option.
- Low-fat or fat-free dressings: Check labels for added sugars and sodium.
- Mustard-based dressings: A good alternative to creamy dressings.

Sample Heart-Healthy Salads

- Grilled chicken salad with mixed greens, avocado, cherry tomatoes, and a balsamic vinaigrette.
- Salmon salad with quinoa, cucumber, red onion, and a dill dressing.
- Tofu salad with edamame, carrots, bell peppers, and a ginger-soy dressing.
- Mediterranean salad with chickpeas, feta cheese, olives, and a lemon-tahini dressing.

Remember to balance your salad with other components of a healthy diet to ensure you're getting all the necessary nutrients.

Soups: A Heart-Healthy Comfort Food

Soups are not only comforting but also a fantastic way to incorporate essential nutrients into your diet. Here are some heart-healthy soup options:

Heart-Healthy Soup Ingredients
- Lean protein: Chicken, turkey, fish, or beans.
- Whole grains: Brown rice, quinoa, or barley.
- Vegetables: A variety of colorful vegetables for vitamins, minerals, and fiber.
- Legumes: Lentils, chickpeas, and kidney beans are excellent sources of protein and fiber.
- Low-sodium broth: The base of your soup.

Soup Ideas
- Lentil soup: Packed with fiber and plant-based protein.
- Vegetable-based soups: Explore options like tomato basil, carrot ginger, or butternut squash.
- Chicken noodle soup: A classic comfort food that can be made healthier with whole-grain noodles and plenty of vegetables.
- Bean soups: White bean, black bean, or chili can be hearty and nutritious.
- Fish-based soups: Salmon or tuna chowder can provide omega-3 fatty acids.

Tips for Heart-Healthy Soups

- Limit added sodium: Check soup labels or reduce salt in homemade versions.
- Incorporate healthy fats: A drizzle of olive oil or a sprinkle of nuts can enhance flavor and provide heart-healthy fats.
- Serve with whole-grain bread: For a complete meal.

By choosing heart-healthy ingredients and preparation methods, you can enjoy a warm and nourishing bowl of soup while supporting your cardiovascular health.

Fish and Seafood: Heart-Healthy Powerhouses

Fish and seafood are excellent sources of protein, vitamins, and minerals. They're particularly renowned for their omega-3 fatty acids, which are linked to numerous heart health benefits.

Omega-3 Fatty Acids

These healthy fats can help:
- Lower triglycerides
- Reduce blood pressure
- Decrease the risk of irregular heartbeats
- Reduce inflammation

Best Fish Choices
- Fatty fish: Salmon, mackerel, tuna, sardines, herring, and trout are rich in omega-3s.
- Lean fish: Cod, halibut, and tilapia are lower in fat but still offer protein and other nutrients.

Preparation Tips
- Grilled, baked, or poached: These cooking methods are healthier than frying.
- Limit added sodium: Be mindful of sauces and marinades.
- Portion control: Enjoy fish as part of a balanced meal.

Incorporating Fish into Your Diet

- Fish tacos: With grilled fish, corn tortillas, and fresh toppings.
- Salmon salad: With mixed greens, avocado, and a light vinaigrette.
- Fish stews: A warm and comforting meal packed with nutrients.
- Seafood pasta: A delicious and satisfying dish.

Remember: While fish is generally healthy, it's essential to be aware of mercury levels, especially in larger fish. Pregnant women and young children should consult dietary guidelines.

Vegetarian Options for a Healthy Heart

A vegetarian diet can be incredibly heart-healthy when planned correctly. It's rich in fiber, antioxidants, and plant-based proteins.

Key Nutrients for Vegetarian Heart Health

- Fiber: Found in abundance in fruits, vegetables, whole grains, and legumes.
- Potassium: Essential for blood pressure control, found in bananas, spinach, and sweet potatoes.
- Magnesium: Helps regulate blood pressure, found in nuts, seeds, and whole grains.
- Plant-based protein: Found in lentils, chickpeas, tofu, tempeh, and soy products.

Heart-Healthy Vegetarian Meals

- Lentil soup: Packed with fiber and protein.
- Chickpea curry: A flavorful and satisfying dish.
- Tofu stir-fry: A quick and easy meal with plenty of vegetables.
- Vegetable-based burgers: Made with beans, lentils, or quinoa.
- Quinoa bowls: A versatile base for various toppings.

Tips for Vegetarian Heart Health

- Include a variety of foods: Ensure you're getting a wide range of nutrients.
- Pay attention to iron intake: Good sources include fortified cereals, lentils, and tofu.
- Vitamin B12: Essential for vegetarians, found in fortified foods or supplements.
- Healthy fats: Incorporate avocados, nuts, and seeds into your diet.

By planning your meals carefully, you can enjoy a delicious and heart-healthy vegetarian lifestyle.

Heart-Healthy Desserts

While indulging in sweets is often associated with unhealthy choices, there are plenty of delicious and heart-healthy dessert options.

Key Ingredients for Heart-Healthy Desserts

- Natural sweeteners: Honey, maple syrup, or fruit purees can replace refined sugar.
- Healthy fats: Olive oil, avocados, and nuts offer heart-healthy fats.
- Fiber: Whole grains, fruits, and nuts provide essential fiber.
- Low-fat dairy: Greek yogurt and cottage cheese offer protein and calcium.

Heart-Healthy Dessert Ideas

- Fruit-based desserts: Fresh fruit, fruit sorbets, or baked apples with cinnamon.
- Yogurt parfaits: Combine Greek yogurt with berries, granola, and a drizzle of honey.
- Dark chocolate: Enjoy in moderation, as it contains antioxidants.
- Chia seed pudding: A creamy and nutritious dessert.
- Rice pudding: Made with low-fat milk and sweetened with natural sweeteners.
- Frozen fruit treats: Blend ripe bananas or berries with a touch of Greek yogurt for a refreshing dessert.

Tips for Heart-Healthy Desserts

- Portion control: Even healthy desserts should be enjoyed in moderation.
- Balance: Pair your dessert with a heart-healthy main course.
- Experiment with flavors: Discover new and exciting ways to satisfy your sweet tooth.

By making informed choices, you can enjoy delicious desserts without compromising your heart health.

The Mediterranean diet is more than just a diet; it's a lifestyle emphasizing whole, plant-based foods, healthy fats, and moderate protein intake. It's renowned for its potential to reduce the risk of heart disease, stroke, and type 2 diabetes.

Core Principles of the Mediterranean Diet

- Emphasis on plant-based foods: Fruits, vegetables, whole grains, legumes, nuts, and seeds form the foundation.
- Healthy fats: Olive oil is the primary source of fat.
- Moderate protein: Primarily from fish, poultry, and eggs. Red meat is consumed infrequently.
- Dairy and eggs: Consumed in moderation.
- Wine: Red wine, in moderation, is often included with meals.

Sample Mediterranean Meal Plan

Breakfast:

- Greek yogurt with berries and nuts
- Oatmeal with fruit and a sprinkle of nuts
- Whole-grain toast with avocado and a poached egg

Lunch:

- Lentil soup with whole-grain bread
- Salad with grilled chicken or fish
- Leftovers from a heart-healthy dinner

Dinner:

- Grilled salmon with roasted vegetables
- Chicken stir-fry with brown rice
- Vegetable-packed pasta with shrimp

Snacks:

- Fruits
- Vegetables with hummus
- Nuts and seeds
- Greek yogurt
- Olives

Tips for Success

- Cook at home: This allows you to control ingredients and portion sizes.
- Read food labels: Look for low-sodium and whole-grain options.
- Enjoy meals with others: Social connections are a key part of the Mediterranean lifestyle.
- Regular physical activity: Combine the diet with exercise for optimal health benefits.

Diving Deeper into the Mediterranean Diet

The Mediterranean Diet: A Lifestyle Approach

The Mediterranean diet is more than just a dietary pattern; it's a lifestyle emphasizing balance, enjoyment, and social connections. Let's explore some key aspects in more detail:

The Role of Olive Oil

Olive oil is the cornerstone of the Mediterranean diet. Rich in monounsaturated fats, it offers numerous health benefits.

- Cooking: Use it for sautéing, roasting, and baking.
- Drizzling: Add a finishing touch to salads and soups.
- Marinades: Create flavorful marinades for grilled meats and vegetables.

The Importance of Legumes

Legumes, such as lentils, chickpeas, and beans, are protein-rich and fiber-packed. They contribute to heart health, weight management, and satiety.

- Hummus: A versatile dip or spread made from chickpeas.
- Lentil soup: A hearty and nutritious meal.
- Bean salads: A refreshing and light option.

The Role of Fish

Fish is a vital component of the Mediterranean diet, providing lean protein and omega-3 fatty acids.

- Variety: Incorporate different types of fish into your diet.
- Sustainable choices: Opt for fish caught using sustainable methods.
- Preparation methods: Grill, bake, or poach for healthier options.

The Mediterranean Mindset

Beyond the food, the Mediterranean lifestyle emphasizes:
- Social dining: Sharing meals with family and friends.
- Mindful eating: Paying attention to hunger cues and enjoying food.
- Regular physical activity: Incorporating exercise into daily life.
- Stress management: Prioritizing relaxation and well-being.

By adopting these principles, you can fully embrace the Mediterranean lifestyle and reap its numerous health benefits.

Part 4: Lifestyle for a Healthy Heart

Section 9.1: Ayurveda for a Healthy Heart

Ayurveda, an ancient Indian system of medicine, offers a holistic approach to heart health. It focuses on balancing the body, mind, and spirit for optimal well-being.

Understanding the Ayurvedic Perspective

Ayurveda views the heart as the seat of consciousness and emotions. A healthy heart is essential for overall vitality. Heart health is closely linked to prana (life force) and ojas (immunity).

Lifestyle for a Healthy Heart

- **Diet:**
    - Emphasize fresh, seasonal, and easily digestible foods.
    - Include plenty of fruits, vegetables, and whole grains.
    - Use ghee (clarified butter) in moderation.
    - Avoid heavy, oily, and processed foods.

- **Lifestyle:**
    - Regular exercise like yoga, walking, or tai chi.
    - Prioritize sufficient sleep.
    - Manage stress through meditation and deep breathing.
    - Cultivate a positive outlook.

Ayurvedic Herbs for Heart Health

Ayurveda offers a rich tradition of herbal remedies for heart health. Here's a deeper look:

- Arjuna (Terminalia arjuna): Often considered the "king of heart tonics," Arjuna strengthens the heart muscle, improves cardiac function, and helps maintain healthy cholesterol levels. It's particularly beneficial for conditions like heart failure and arrhythmias.
- Ashwagandha (Withania somnifera): Known as an adaptogen, Ashwagandha helps the body manage stress, which is a significant factor in heart disease. It also supports adrenal function and overall well-being.
- Guggul (Commiphora mukul): Traditionally used to manage cholesterol levels, Guggul helps maintain healthy lipid profiles. It's often combined with other herbs for optimal heart health.
- Brahmi (Bacopa monnieri): While primarily known for its brain-boosting properties, Brahmi also supports overall cardiovascular health by promoting relaxation and reducing stress.
- Triphala: A combination of three fruits, Triphala is a general detoxifier that supports overall health, including heart function.

Note: It's crucial to consult with an Ayurvedic practitioner before starting any herbal supplement. They can determine the appropriate dosage and combination based on your individual needs.

Ayurvedic Treatments

Ayurvedic treatments focus on restoring balance to the body and mind.

- Panchakarma: A comprehensive detoxification process involving five procedures (Vamana, Virechan, Basti, Nasya, and Shirodhara). It helps eliminate toxins from the body, improving overall health, including heart function.

- Abhyanga: This full-body massage using warm herbal oils relaxes the muscles, improves circulation, and promotes sleep.

- Shirodhara: A continuous stream of warm oil is poured onto the forehead to calm the mind and reduce stress.

- Diet and Lifestyle: As mentioned earlier, Ayurveda emphasizes a balanced diet, regular exercise, and stress management as essential components of heart health.

Remember: These treatments should be administered by trained professionals in a supervised setting.

Aromatherapy for a Healthy Heart

Aromatherapy, the therapeutic use of essential oils, can indirectly support heart health by promoting relaxation and reducing stress. While it's not a direct treatment for heart disease, it can complement other heart-healthy practices.

Essential Oils for Heart Health
- Lavender: Known for its calming properties, lavender can help reduce stress and anxiety, which can positively impact heart health.
- Rose: Like lavender, rose oil has calming effects and may help lower blood pressure.
- Eucalyptus: Some studies suggest eucalyptus oil can lower blood pressure.
- Bergamot: This citrus oil has a calming effect and may help reduce anxiety.
- Ylang-ylang: Known for its balancing properties, ylang-ylang can help regulate blood pressure and heart rate.

Ways to Use Essential Oils
- Inhalation: Directly inhale the aroma from the bottle or use a diffuser.
- Massage: Dilute a few drops of essential oil in a carrier oil (like coconut or almond oil) and massage into the chest or temples.
- Bath: Add a few drops of essential oil to a warm bath for relaxation.

Section 9.2: Aromatherapy for a Healthy Heart

Important Considerations

- Always dilute essential oils before applying them to the skin.
- Avoid using essential oils if you have allergies or sensitivities.
- Consult with a healthcare professional before using essential oils if you have underlying health conditions.

Aromatherapy should be considered a complementary approach to heart health, not a replacement for medical treatment. It's essential to maintain a healthy lifestyle, including diet, exercise, and stress management, for optimal heart health.

While it's essential to focus on a balanced diet and lifestyle for heart health, certain plants can offer additional support.

Herbs with Heart-Healthy Properties

While these herbs have shown promise in supporting heart health, it's crucial to approach them as complementary to a healthy lifestyle and medical treatment, not as replacements.

Hawthorn Berry (Crataegus spp.)

- How it works: Contains flavonoids that relax blood vessels, improve blood flow, and strengthen the heart muscle.
- Potential benefits: May help with mild heart failure, angina, and arrhythmias.
- Cautions: Can interact with certain heart medications.

Garlic (Allium sativum)

- How it works: Contains compounds like allicin that have anti-inflammatory and blood-thinning properties.
- Potential benefits: Lowers blood pressure, reduces cholesterol levels, and inhibits platelet aggregation.
- Cautions: Can interact with blood-thinning medications.

Ginkgo Biloba

- How it works: Improves blood circulation by dilating blood vessels.
- Potential benefits: May help with memory and cognitive function, but its effects on heart health are less clear.
- Cautions: Can interact with blood-thinning medications and anti-seizure drugs.

Cayenne Pepper (Capsicum annuum)

- How it works: Contains capsaicin, which can help lower blood pressure by dilating blood vessels.
- Potential benefits: May also aid digestion and metabolism.
- Cautions: Use with caution if you have stomach ulcers or other digestive issues.

Remember, it's crucial to consult with a healthcare provider before starting any new supplements, especially if you have underlying health conditions or are taking medications.

Heart-Healthy Foods

Incorporating these plant-based foods into your diet can contribute to overall heart health:

- Leafy Green Vegetables: Rich in vitamins, minerals, and antioxidants.
- Berries: Packed with antioxidants and fiber.
- Whole Grains: Provide essential nutrients and fiber.
- Nuts and Seeds: Offer healthy fats, fiber, and plant-based protein.
- Avocados: A good source of heart-healthy monounsaturated fats.

Important Note

While these plants offer potential benefits, it's essential to consult with a healthcare provider before starting any new supplements or making significant dietary changes.

A meditation program is a structured approach to cultivating mindfulness and inner peace. It can vary widely in length, intensity, and focus, but typically involves regular practice and guidance.

Key Components of a Meditation Program

- Mindfulness Techniques: Core practices like focused attention, body scan, and loving-kindness meditation.
- Breath Awareness: Learning to observe and regulate your breath.
- Posture: Proper sitting or lying down positions for comfort and focus.
- Guided Meditation: Using audio or visual cues to facilitate deeper states of relaxation.
- Silent Meditation: Practicing without external guidance.
- Mindful Movement: Incorporating physical activities like yoga or tai chi.

Popular Meditation Programs

- Mindfulness-Based Stress Reduction (MBSR): Focuses on reducing stress and improving overall well-being.
- Mindfulness-Based Cognitive Therapy (MBCT): Specifically designed for individuals with depression.
- Transcendental Meditation (TM): Uses a specific mantra to promote relaxation and inner peace.
- Vipassana Meditation: Emphasizes insight into the nature of reality through observation of bodily sensations.

Creating Your Own Meditation Program

- Set Clear Goals: Determine what you hope to achieve through meditation (e.g., stress reduction, increased focus, emotional balance).
- Choose a Suitable Time: Find a quiet space and time of day that works best for you.
- Start Slowly: Begin with short meditation sessions and gradually increase duration.
- Experiment with Techniques: Try different meditation styles to find what resonates with you.
- Be Consistent: Regular practice is key to experiencing benefits.
- Find a Community: Consider joining a meditation group or finding a meditation teacher for support.

Benefits of Meditation

- Reduced stress and anxiety
- Improved focus and concentration
- Enhanced emotional regulation
- Increased self-awareness
- Better sleep quality
- Strengthned immune system

Yoga for Heart Health

Yoga offers a holistic approach to improving heart health by combining physical postures, breathing exercises, and meditation.

How Yoga Benefits the Heart

- Reduces stress: Stress is a major contributor to heart disease. Yoga helps manage stress through relaxation techniques and mindfulness.
- Lowers blood pressure: Regular yoga practice can help reduce high blood pressure.
- Improves circulation: Certain yoga poses enhance blood flow throughout the body.
- Increases lung capacity: Deeper breathing exercises improve oxygen intake.
- Builds strength and flexibility: Stronger heart muscles and increased flexibility contribute to overall heart health.

Yoga Poses for Heart Health

While all yoga poses offer benefits, certain poses are particularly beneficial for heart health:

- Tadasana (Mountain Pose): Improves posture, balance, and grounding.
- Vrikshasana (Tree Pose): Enhances balance and focus, strengthening the legs.

- Utkatasana (Chair Pose): Builds lower body strength and improves cardiovascular health.
- Adho Mukha Svanasana (Downward-Facing Dog): Inverts the body, improving blood circulation and calming the mind.
- Bhujangasana (Cobra Pose): Strengthens the spine, chest, and heart.
- Savasana (Corpse Pose): Deep relaxation and stress reduction.

Incorporating Yoga into Your Routine

- Start slowly: Begin with gentle yoga classes and gradually increase intensity.
- Find a qualified teacher: A certified yoga instructor can provide guidance and support.
- Regular practice: Aim for at least 20-30 minutes of yoga most days of the week.
- Listen to your body: Pay attention to your physical limitations and avoid overexertion.

Remember, yoga is a complementary approach to heart health. It should be combined with a healthy diet, regular exercise, and medical supervision if necessary.

Chapter 10: Exercise Routine for Cardiovascular Fitness

Regular cardiovascular exercise is essential for a healthy heart. It strengthens the heart muscle, improves circulation, and helps manage conditions like high blood pressure and cholesterol.

Types of Cardiovascular Exercise

- Aerobic exercises: These elevate your heart rate and breathing for an extended period. Examples include:
  - Running or jogging
  - Swimming
  - Cycling
  - Dancing
  - Walking briskly
  - Hiking
  - Rowing
- Interval training: Alternates between short bursts of high-intensity exercise and periods of rest.
- Circuit training: Involves performing a series of exercises with minimal rest between them.

Building a Cardiovascular Workout Routine

- Start gradually: Begin with low-intensity exercises and gradually increase duration and intensity.
- Warm-up: Engage in light activity like walking or jogging for a few minutes before starting your workout.
- Cool-down: Gradually reduce intensity with activities like stretching or walking.
- Variety: Incorporate different types of exercise to prevent boredom and challenge your body.

Chapter 10: Exercise Routine for Cardiovascular Fitness

- Consistency: Aim for at least 150 minutes of moderate-intensity exercise or 75 minutes of vigorous-intensity exercise per week.

Sample Workout Routine

Beginner:
- Start with 30 minutes of brisk walking, 3 times a week.
- Gradually increase duration and intensity.

Intermediate:
- Combine 30 minutes of running or swimming with strength training twice a week.
- Incorporate interval training sessions.

Advanced:
- Aim for 45-60 minutes of high-intensity workouts, 3-4 times per week.
- Include cross-training activities like cycling or swimming.

Important Considerations

- Listen to your body: Pay attention to any pain or discomfort.
- Stay hydrated: Drink plenty of water before, during, and after exercise.
- Wear appropriate footwear: Choose shoes designed for your chosen activity.
- Consult your doctor: If you have underlying health conditions.

Remember, consistency is key. Find activities you enjoy and make exercise a regular part of your lifestyle.

Chapter 11: Physical Activity for Cardiovascular System Health

Regular physical activity is a cornerstone of heart health. It helps strengthen the heart muscle, improve circulation, and reduce the risk of heart disease.

Types of Physical Activity

- Aerobic exercise: This increases heart rate and breathing, improving cardiovascular endurance. Examples include:
    - Walking, jogging, running
    - Swimming, water aerobics
    - Cycling, stationary cycling
    - Dancing
    - Rowing
- Strength training: Builds muscle mass and improves metabolism.
    - Weightlifting
    - Bodyweight exercises (push-ups, squats, lunges)
    - Resistance band exercises
- Flexibility exercises: Improves range of motion and reduces muscle tension.
    - Yoga
    - Stretching

How Much Physical Activity?

- Aim for at least 150 minutes of moderate-intensity aerobic activity or 75 minutes of vigorous-intensity aerobic activity per week.
- Incorporate strength training exercises at least twice a week.

Chapter 11: Physical Activity for Cardiovascular System Health

Incorporate strength training exercises at least twice a week.

Benefits of Physical Activity for the Heart

- Reduces risk of heart disease: Regular exercise lowers blood pressure, cholesterol levels, and the risk of blood clots.
- Improves heart function: Strengthens the heart muscle, increasing its pumping efficiency.
- Controls weight: Helps maintain a healthy weight, reducing strain on the heart.
- Reduces stress: Physical activity can help manage stress levels.
- Boosts mood: Releases endorphins, which can improve mood and overall well-being.

Tips for Getting Started

- Start slowly: Begin with short workouts and gradually increase duration and intensity.
- Find activities you enjoy: This will make it easier to stick with your exercise routine.
- Vary your workouts: This prevents boredom and challenges different muscle groups.
- Listen to your body: Pay attention to any pain or discomfort.
- Make it a habit: Schedule exercise into your daily routine

Chapter 12: The Simple Heart Cure Food List

While the specific foods included in Dr. Crandall's "Simple Heart Cure Food List" may vary, the core principles align with a heart-healthy diet. Here's a general overview of food groups to prioritize:

Heart-Healthy Food Groups
- Fruits and vegetables: Rich in vitamins, minerals, and fiber. Aim for a variety of colors.
- Whole grains: Provide sustained energy and fiber. Examples include brown rice, quinoa, whole-wheat bread, and oats.
- Lean proteins: Opt for sources like poultry, fish, beans, lentils, and tofu.
- Healthy fats: Found in avocados, nuts, seeds, and olive oil.
- Low-fat dairy: Choose Greek yogurt or low-fat milk for calcium and protein.

Fruits and Vegetables
- Leafy greens: spinach, kale, collard greens
- Berries: strawberries, blueberries, raspberries
- Citrus fruits: oranges, grapefruits, lemons
- Apples, bananas, pears
- Tomatoes, carrots, broccoli, peppers

Whole Grains
- Brown rice
- Quinoa
- Oatmeal
- Whole-wheat bread
- Whole-grain pasta

Chapter 12: The Simple Heart Cure Food List

Lean Proteins
- Fish: salmon, tuna, mackerel
- Poultry: chicken, turkey
- Beans and legumes: lentils, chickpeas, kidney beans
- Tofu and tempeh
- Eggs

Healthy Fats
- Olive oil
- Avocados
- Nuts and seeds: almonds, walnuts, chia seeds, flaxseeds

Low-Fat Dairy
- Greek yogurt
- Low-fat milk and cheese

Other Heart-Healthy Foods
- Garlic
- Oats
- Soy products
- Dark chocolate (in moderation)

Foods to Limit or Avoid
- Processed foods: High in sodium, unhealthy fats, and added sugars.
- Red meat: Consume in moderation due to its higher saturated fat content.
- Refined grains: Opt for whole-grain alternatives.
- Excessive sugar and sugary drinks: Contribute to weight gain and other health issues.

Chapter 12: The Simple Heart Cure Food List

- Trans fats: Found in processed foods and harmful to heart health.

Sample Heart-Healthy Meal
- Breakfast: Oatmeal with berries and nuts, or Greek yogurt with honey and fruit.
- Lunch: Salad with grilled chicken or fish, or a lentil soup with whole-grain bread.
- Dinner: Salmon with roasted vegetables, or whole-grain pasta with marinara sauce and lean protein.
- Snacks: Fruits, vegetables, nuts, or seeds.

Remember: This is a general guideline. Individual needs may vary. It's essential to consult with a healthcare professional for personalized dietary advice.

Part 5: Healing Strategies

Part 5: Healing Strategies
Chapter 13: Good Habits for a Healthy Heart
Section 13.1: Setting Realistic Goals

Setting achievable goals is crucial for improving heart health. Here's how to create realistic and effective targets:

Understand Your Starting Point

- Assess your current health: Review your blood pressure, cholesterol levels, and overall fitness.
- Identify areas for improvement: Determine which areas need the most attention, such as diet, exercise, or stress management.

Set Specific, Measurable, Achievable, Relevant, and Time-bound (SMART) Goals

- Be specific: Instead of "eat healthier," aim for "increase fruit and vegetable intake to five servings per day."
- Make it measurable: Track your progress with a food diary or fitness tracker.
- Set achievable goals: Start with small, manageable steps and gradually increase challenges.
- Ensure relevance: Choose goals that align with your overall health and lifestyle.
- Establish a timeline: Set deadlines for achieving your goals.

Examples of Realistic Goals

- Diet: Reduce sodium intake by 500mg per day, incorporate two servings of fish per week.
- Exercise: Walk for 30 minutes, five days a week, or join a gym.
- Weight management: Lose 5% of body weight in three months.

- Stress management: Practice meditation or yoga for 10 minutes daily.
- Blood pressure control: Reduce blood pressure by 10 points in three months.

Celebrate Successes
- Acknowledge your achievements: Reward yourself for reaching milestones.
- Stay motivated: Celebrate small wins to maintain enthusiasm.

Remember: It's essential to be patient and kind to yourself. Progress takes time, and setbacks are normal. Focus on creating sustainable lifestyle changes rather than quick fixes.

Part 5: Healing Strategies
Chapter 13: Good Habits for a Healthy Heart
Section 13.2: Creating a Plan

A heart-healthy lifestyle involves a combination of diet, exercise, stress management, and regular check-ups. Here's a general outline to get you started:

Diet

- Prioritize whole foods: Focus on fruits, vegetables, whole grains, lean proteins, and healthy fats.
- Limit processed foods: Reduce intake of sugary drinks, fast food, and highly processed snacks.
- Control portion sizes: Be mindful of serving sizes to maintain a healthy weight.
- Read food labels: Pay attention to sodium, saturated fat, and added sugar content.

Exercise

- Aim for 150 minutes of moderate-intensity exercise or 75 minutes of vigorous-intensity exercise per week.
- Incorporate strength training: Build muscle to boost metabolism.
- Find activities you enjoy: This will make it easier to stick to your exercise routine.

Stress Management

- Practice relaxation techniques: Try meditation, deep breathing, or yoga.
- Get enough sleep: Aim for 7-9 hours of quality sleep per night.
- Build a strong support system: Spend time with loved ones and engage in social activities.

Regular Check-ups

- Monitor blood pressure, cholesterol, and blood sugar levels.
- Schedule regular appointments with your healthcare provider.

Additional Tips

- Quit smoking: Smoking significantly increases heart disease risk.
- Limit alcohol consumption: Excessive alcohol can harm your heart.
- Stay hydrated: Drink plenty of water throughout the day.

Remember: This is a general guideline. Individual needs may vary. It's essential to consult with a healthcare professional for personalized advice

Educating Yourself About Heart Health

Understanding heart health is crucial for preventing and managing cardiovascular disease. Here are key areas to focus on:

Understanding Heart Disease
- Types of heart disease: Learn about different types like coronary artery disease, heart failure, arrhythmias, and valvular heart disease.
- Risk factors: Understand modifiable and non-modifiable risk factors (e.g., smoking, high blood pressure, cholesterol, diabetes, family history).
- Symptoms: Recognize warning signs of a heart attack or stroke.

Healthy Lifestyle Choices
- Diet: Learn about heart-healthy foods, portion control, and reading food labels.
- Exercise: Understand the importance of both aerobic and strength training.
- Weight management: The connection between weight and heart health.
- Stress management: Techniques for reducing stress and its impact on the heart.
- Sleep: The role of sleep in heart health.

Medical Check-ups and Screenings

- Importance of regular check-ups: Blood pressure, cholesterol, and blood sugar monitoring.
- Recommended screenings: Discuss appropriate screenings with your doctor (e.g., electrocardiogram, echocardiogram).

Medications and Treatments

- Understanding heart medications: How they work and potential side effects.
- Treatment options: Learn about procedures like angioplasty, stents, and bypass surgery.

Resources

- Reliable sources: Utilize reputable organizations like the American Heart Association, Mayo Clinic, and National Institutes of Health.
- Online information: Be cautious about the credibility of online sources.
- Consult your doctor: Discuss any concerns or questions with your healthcare provider.

By educating yourself about heart health, you can take proactive steps to protect your heart and enjoy a healthier life.

While lifestyle changes and education are crucial for heart health, sometimes professional guidance is necessary. Here's when to consider seeking professional help:

Reasons to Consult a Healthcare Professional

- Persistent symptoms: If you experience chest pain, shortness of breath, or other concerning symptoms.
- Family history of heart disease: Increased risk might require closer monitoring.
- Risk factors: If you have multiple risk factors like high blood pressure, diabetes, or obesity.
- Medication management: Need help understanding or managing heart medications.
- Lifestyle challenges: Difficulty making significant lifestyle changes.

Types of Healthcare Professionals

- Cardiologist: A specialist in heart conditions.
- Primary care physician: General healthcare provider who can monitor overall health and refer to specialists.
- Registered dietitian: Can provide personalized dietary advice.
- Mental health professional: Can help manage stress and anxiety.

Finding the Right Professional

- Insurance coverage: Check if your insurance covers specific healthcare providers.
- Recommendations: Ask friends, family, or your primary care physician for referrals.
- Credentials and experience: Look for board-certified professionals with relevant experience.

Building a Strong Partnership

- Open communication: Be honest about your health concerns and lifestyle.
- Ask questions: Don't hesitate to seek clarification or additional information.
- Adherence to treatment plan: Follow your doctor's recommendations consistently.

By working closely with healthcare professionals, you can develop a comprehensive plan to protect your heart health.

Stress is a common experience, but chronic stress can significantly impact heart health. Understanding stress and implementing effective management techniques are crucial for maintaining a healthy heart.

The Link Between Stress and Heart Health

Chronic stress triggers the body's "fight-or-flight" response, leading to:
- Increased heart rate and blood pressure
- Hormonal imbalances
- Weakened immune system
- Increased risk of heart disease, stroke, and heart attack

Stress Management Techniques
- Mindfulness and Meditation: These practices help reduce stress by focusing on the present moment.
- Deep Breathing: Simple yet effective, deep breathing can lower blood pressure and promote relaxation.
- Yoga and Tai Chi: Combining physical movement with mindfulness, these practices offer stress relief.
- Progressive Muscle Relaxation: Focusing on relaxing different muscle groups can reduce tension.
- Time Management: Effective time management can reduce feelings of overwhelm and stress.
- Social Support: Building strong relationships can provide emotional support and reduce stress.
- Physical Activity: Regular exercise helps manage stress and improve overall health.

Incorporating Stress Management into Daily Life

- Identify stressors: Understand what triggers stress in your life.
- Set realistic goals: Avoid overcommitting yourself.
- Prioritize tasks: Focus on important tasks and delegate when possible.
- Take breaks: Schedule short breaks throughout the day to relax and recharge.
- Practice self-care: Engage in activities you enjoy, such as hobbies or spending time in nature.

By implementing these strategies, you can significantly reduce stress levels and improve your heart health.

The Importance of Sleep for Heart Health

Sleep is often overlooked as a crucial component of overall health, but it plays a significant role in heart health.

How Sleep Affects Your Heart

- Regulates Blood Pressure: Sleep helps maintain a healthy blood pressure level. Disrupted sleep can contribute to hypertension.
- Reduces Stress Hormones: During sleep, the body releases hormones that help manage stress. Insufficient sleep can elevate stress hormones, negatively impacting heart health.
- Supports Immune Function: Sleep is essential for a strong immune system, which helps protect against heart disease.
- Aids in Blood Sugar Control: Sleep helps regulate blood sugar levels, reducing the risk of diabetes, a major heart disease risk factor.
- Promotes Heart Repair: The body undergoes repair and regeneration processes during sleep, including heart tissue.

Tips for Better Sleep

- Consistent Sleep Schedule: Try to go to bed and wake up at the same time each day, even on weekends.
- Create a Sleep-Conducive Environment: Ensure your bedroom is dark, quiet, and cool.
- Limit Screen Time: The blue light emitted by electronic devices can interfere with sleep.

- Manage Stress: Incorporate relaxation techniques like meditation or deep breathing before bed.
- Watch Your Diet: Avoid heavy meals, caffeine, and alcohol close to bedtime.
- Regular Exercise: Physical activity can improve sleep quality, but avoid intense workouts right before bed.

By prioritizing sleep, you can significantly enhance your overall well-being and reduce the risk of heart disease.

www.ingramcontent.com/pod-product-compliance
Lightning Source LLC
Chambersburg PA
CBHW070738250726
48662CB00004B/1577